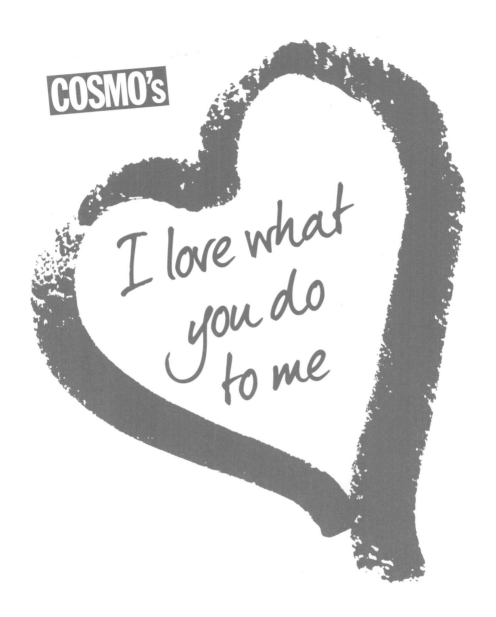

COSMO's

I love what you do to me

HEARST BOOKS
New York

HEARST BOOKS
New York

An Imprint of Sterling Publishing
387 Park Avenue South
New York, NY 10016

Illustrations on pages 41–51 by Bo Lundberg

ISBN 978-1-61837-160-7

Distributed in Canada by Sterling Publishing
c/o Canadian Manda Group, 165 Dufferin Street
Toronto, Ontario, Canada M6K 3H6
Distributed in the United Kingdom by GMC Distribution Services
Castle Place, 166 High Street, Lewes, East Sussex, England BN7 1XU
Distributed in Australia by Capricorn Link (Australia) Pty. Ltd.
P.O. Box 704, Windsor, NSW 2756, Australia

For information about custom editions, special sales, and premium and
corporate purchases, please contact Sterling Special Sales at 800-805-
5489 or specialsales@sterlingpublishing.com.

Manufactured in China

2 4 6 8 10 9 7 5 3 1

www.sterlingpublishing.com

CONTENTS

GETTING FRISKY (FOREPLAY!)

LET'S TALK ABOUT SEX, BABY

HOW ABOUT SOME SEXTRAS?

GETTING FRISKY (FOREPLAY!)

CHAPTER 1

HIS & HER SEX DRIVES

Here's the deal: Throughout this chapter, you'll take a few quizzes about yourselves and each other. Then you'll compare notes to see how well you match up. Ready, set, go!

FOR HER

WHAT'S YOUR SEX STYLE?

1. If we were to look into your nightstand drawer, we'd be most likely to find:

  a. Your journal, a book light, and some aspirin.
  b. Sultry perfume, breath mints, and a sleep mask you may or may not have used once to blindfold your guy.
  c. Condoms, flavored lube, and a 24-pack of spare batteries for your numerous toys.

FOR HIM

WHAT'S HER SEX STYLE?

1. If you were to look into her nightstand drawer, you'd probably find:

  a. Her journal, a book light, and some aspirin.
  b. Her sultry perfume, breath mints, and a sleep mask she's used to blindfold you.
  c. Condoms, flavored lube, and a 24-pack of spare batteries for your numerous toys.

2. You want to rev up your guy with a naughty text. What does it say?

a. Nothing...the attached pic of your cleavage is worth a thousand words.

b. "Can't wait 2 see u 2nite."

c. "Wanna guess if I have panties on right now?"

3. The craziest place you would ever have sex is:

a. In the dressing room of a big (but mostly deserted) store.

b. In a crowded movie theater.

c. In a car…as long as the windows are steamed up and you're feeling really adventurous.

4. When you want some ideas to spice things up, you go to:

a. No one. You're perfectly happy with positions you've already tried, thanks.

b. The animalistic orgy scenes in season two of *True Blood*.

c. *Cosmo*, of course.

5. Post-sex, you're used to hearing:

a. "Mmm, that was nice."

b. Deep breathing—your man usually falls asleep instantly.

c. "That was f#$%ing amazing."

2. When she sends you a naughty text before your date night, it says:

a. Nothing. It's just a picture of her cleavage.

b. "Can't wait to see you tonight."

c. "Wanna guess if I have panties on right now?"

3. The craziest place you think she'd ever want to have sex is:

a. In the dressing room of a big (but mostly deserted) store.

b. In a crowded movie theater.

c. In a car…as long as the windows are steamed up and she's feeling adventurous.

4. When she wants ideas to spice things up in bed, she turns to:

a. No one. She's perfectly happy with the positions she's already tried, thanks.

b. The animalistic orgy scenes in *True Blood*.

c. *Cosmo*, of course.

5. Post-sex, you usually say to her:

a. "Mmm, that was nice."

b. Nothing—you fall asleep right away.

c. "That was f#$%ing amazing."

7 TO 10 POINTS: COY CUTIE

You love nooky as much as the next girl, but you're not about to initiate anything outside your comfort zone. "Men can interpret an unwillingness to try new things as rejection," says Regina Lynn, author of *Sexier Sex*. But you may be missing out on some major fun! If you don't want to swap positions as often as you do your days-of-the-week undies, stick to baby steps. Instead of having sex in public places (way too risky!), try getting busy in your backyard late at night.

4 TO 6 POINTS: VA-VA-VIXEN

Any dude who lands in your bed is lucky. Since you appreciate aggressive, rowdy nights as well as soft-'n'-slow ones, you have the perfect mix of mattress moves to max out your pleasure (and his). "You like to switch it up but are also balanced enough to realize that the best sex doesn't necessarily come from trying something new every time," says sexologist Logan Levkoff, PhD. "It's about being in tune with how you and your partner feel in the moment and doing something that matches that."

0 TO 3 POINTS: OVER-THE-TOP TEMPTRESS

No one's stopping you when you're in action, but your guy may not be as into Cirque du Soleil–worthy routines as you are. "Despite what you might expect, not all men want to do everything humanly possible," Levkoff says. Plus, having tried-and-true standbys to revisit can build romantic intimacy—so decide together what those are instead of always trying to top your last feat!

HOW BARE DO YOU DARE?

Cosmo created a quiz to determine your "nude attitude." Circle your answers, then let your man see the results so he knows how you feel about your body in the buff.

1. **You and your friends are on a lingerie excursion. First item up for grabs? A sequined thong. Your response:**
   a. No way—you want as much cotton coverage as possible. Live by the Loom, die by the Loom.
   b. Thong, schmong. Why not save money and go naked (as always)?
   c. Ante up. Nothing like a little undercover naughtiness to spice up your day.

2. **After working out, your locker room routine is to:**
   a. Change out of your sweaty clothes in the bathroom stall so no one gets a glimpse of your goodies.
   b. Quickly hop out of the shower and avoid conversation until you've put on your bra and panties.
   c. Stretch, apply a full face of makeup, and discuss the latest episode of *Scandal* with your neighbors—au naturel.

3. **You take the day to go swimsuit shopping and are forced to change in a communal dressing room. You:**
   a. Happily strip, then ask fellow shoppers, "Do my nipples look weird to you?"
   b. Undress as if you were alone but keep your eyes on your own prizes.
   c. Try the suit on over your regular clothes. You're not about to show your skin to a bunch of complete strangers.

4. **You're about to do serious sack time with your new man. While he preps the bed, you:**
   a. Unleash your assets and purr, "Feast your eyes on these babies!"
   b. Emerge in your favorite cotton jammies. When things get really crazy, you'll let him undo the flap.
   c. Peel off your clothes to reveal your sexiest bra and panty set. He can take it from there.

5. Your sister tells you that she and her husband are going on a nudist retreat. You:

  a. Reply, "That's great!" and then call your mom to let her know that she raised a pervert.

  b. Are happy for her—just as long as you don't have to sit through a slide show when they come back.

  c. Scoff, "Who needs a retreat?" You do the backyard in the buff whenever the mood strikes you.

6. After one too many drinks at a party, the host suggests a midnight skinny-dip. You:

  a. Feign a communicable disease and make tracks to the nearest exit.

  b. Cheer them on, but keep your clothes on and your dignity intact.

  c. Streak to the pool screaming, "Last one in is a rotten egg!"

7. You're watching an indie flick with a first date when the lead actor drops his pants and gives the audience the full monty. You:

  a. Rush to the candy counter for more Skittles—whether you're hungry for them or not.

  b. Cringe a little and feel thankful that the dim lights cover your momentary blushing.

  c. Remark loudly, "I've seen bigger."

8. While visiting your parents, you unexpectedly walk in on your dad—completely naked. You:

  a. Commence therapy. Seeing the equipment of your origin is too much for you to endure without the help of a trained professional.

  b. Immediately shut the door and call out an apology. Yes, going through life without seeing your father's "family tree" would have been ideal, but you can put it behind you.

  c. Aren't a bit fazed. You've seen *plenty* of naked men before.

9. Your best friend confides in you that she worked as a topless dancer to earn cash in college. You:

  a. Pity her. The real money was in the bottomless industry.

  b. Are appalled. Why didn't she just sell crack to schoolchildren?

  c. Probe her for a few details but then drop the topic. The past is in the past.

10. After a dinner party with friends, someone suggests a game of strip poker. You:

  a. Lose on purpose. When you're nude, *everybody* wins.
  b. Agree, but not before you put your coat, gloves, and hat back on.
  c. Go for it—just as long as you don't have to go past your skivvies.

ANSWER KEY

1. A-0; B-2; C-1   **2.** A-0; B-1; C-2   **3.** A-2; B-1; C-0
4. A-2; B-0; C-1   **5.** A-0; B-1; C-2   **6.** A-0; B-1; C-2
7. A-0; B-1; C-2   **8.** A-0; B-1; C-2   **9.** A-2; B-0; C-1

Add up your points and see where you netted out!

---

16 TO 20 POINTS: BRAZEN BARE-ASS

An orangutan has more inhibitions than you. Happy to share your wares at the slightest provocation, your unabashed behavior puts you somewhere between *Penthouse* and *National Geographic*. "You flaunt your outside because you're afraid of what's on the inside," says Katie Arons, author of *Sexy at Any Size*. That's not to say that pride in one's appearance is a mark against you. But if bare-assed is the only way you can bear to be, then your au naturel actions reveal more about you than your butt cheeks. "As a child, you may not have been valued on the basis of your talents and abilities, so you looked to your appearance to give you the recognition that you needed," says Arons. Add that to the thrill you got by shocking others with your exhibitionism and voilà: A flesh-flaunting fetish was born. How can you break from your "dare to bare" mentality? "The key is to base your worth on something other than your appearance," says Arons. Set goals in life that reflect something other than what you see in the mirror. People will pay attention to you when you're wearing more than your bra and panties if you say or do something worthwhile.

8 TO 15 POINTS: SEMI-BUFF BABE

You're no nude prude—you're not afraid to take it off when the time is right. See, in your eyes, an okay body image isn't necessarily equated with swiveling around a pole in your birthday suit. You have an appreciation of the human body in all its fleshy forms, yes, but you still know where to draw the line between Amish and *oh my gosh!* "Your parents probably accepted you as is," says Arons, and as a result, you've been able to dodge the confidence killers that can sideswipe a healthy self-image but haven't had to resort to buck-naked behavior to get noticed. Just maintain that balance between your self-image and the mirror image and you'll keep liking what you see both in and out of your clothes.

0 TO 7 POINTS: BUTTONED-UP BORE

No nude is good nude as far as you're concerned. You see shedding clothes as shameful rather than accepting nakedness as a normal, natural human state, and with your skewed view comes a plethora of problems involving body image, sexuality, and human nature in general. In fact, just the thought of having to take it off can send you into puritanical panic, fearful that someone other than your cat might see you in your God-given splendor. That's not to say you should be plastering your boobs on a billboard, but your reluctance to reveal can be almost as stifling as the turtleneck pajama set you wear to bed. "Some people have a negative body image because their self-perception isn't in tune with reality," says Monica Ramirez Basco, PhD, author of *Never Good Enough: Freeing Yourself from the Chains of Perfectionism*, and others associate it solely with sex. To improve your nude attitude, stop thinking of nakedness as dirty and start thinking of it as simply part of the package of being a person. And if a beat-up body image is making you cover up, take a good look around you. "In the real world, most women don't fit those cookie-cutter images you see in the media," says Arons. "So why should you be expected to meet such strict standards?" Once you accept others in all stages of undress, you'll become as comfortable in your skin as you are in that flannel jumper.

COSMO COUPLES QUIZ 1

Solid twosomes have strong bonds. Fill out this simple questionnaire to determine how synced up you are with each other outside the bedroom—it can tell you a lot about how you connect between the sheets.

Here's how it works: Write down your answers to each question in the left-hand column, then ask your man how he thinks you responded. After that, have him fill out the right-hand column and ask you to guess how he answered. If each of you gets at least seven right, it means you're enviably fused.

FOR HER	FOR HIM
1. Where's my ideal vacation spot?	1. What do I see myself doing in 10 years?
2. Who's my closest friend?	2. If forced, would I rather be made to dance or sing in public?
3. Who's my celebrity crush?	3. Who's my celebrity crush?
4. What's my least favorite food?	4. If I had to switch jobs with one of my friends, who would it be?

FOR HER	FOR HIM
5. What ice-cream flavor do I crave?	5. How do I like my steak done?
6. Where were we the first time we had sex?	6. What genre of movie do I usually want to watch?
7. What's my favorite gift you've ever given me?	7. Which of my body parts do I like the most?
8. What form of exercise do I enjoy most?	8. Who in my family do I call first with good news?
9. Which of my body parts do I like the most?	9. Would I pick fame or fortune?
10. What genre of movie do I usually want to watch?	10. Where am I most comfortable: in the city or the country?
TOTAL CORRECT:	TOTAL CORRECT:

COSMO COUPLES QUIZ 2

These "would you rather?" questions might seem totally random, but your choices uncover a whole lot about your respective appetites for adventure.

WOULD YOU RATHER... **...order an appetizer?** OR **...order dessert?**

○ ME ○ YOU ○ ME ○ YOU

You don't feel the need to rush to the entrée, and the same holds true in your relationship. Instead of thinking about what milestone you should be reaching next— saying *I love you,* moving in together—you stay focused on the now and want to be with someone who is able to do the same.

You savor your partner just like you would a piece of cake: taking in and appreciating everything that makes that person special to you. Are you dating someone like this? Stick a note in their wallet telling them one little thing they do that drives you crazy with lust.

WOULD YOU RATHER... **...go on an adventurous trip** OR **...veg out at a tropical resort?**

○ ME ○ YOU ○ ME ○ YOU

You need your significant other to be your partner in crime— someone who's always up for trying new things. If you are involved with someone like this, find ways to incorporate fun, silly events into your relationship (think waking up to eat ice cream in the middle of the night or spending the day at an arcade).

A calm and relaxing atmosphere is of the utmost importance to you. You always remain levelheaded and don't let emotions or drama rule your life. If you're dating this type, try to stay cool during stressful times and in fights. Screaming and yelling will just make him or her shut down and stop listening to you.

WOULD YOU RATHER...

...be a celebrity	OR	...be a well-known author

○ **ME** ○ **YOU**   ○ **ME** ○ **YOU**

You live for grand, movie-style romantic gestures and show your love through things like flowers and unexpected gifts. Is this your partner? Tell them to get all dressed up and then head out to dinner at a fancy restaurant. They'll adore being made to feel like Hollywood royalty.

Your ultimate goal in a relationship is to have the other person consider you invaluable, and you go out of your way to make them feel the same. Words are really important to this person. If you're with this type, make sure to describe exactly what it is about being with them that you love so much.

WOULD YOU RATHER...

...take a short plane trip	OR	...drive there?

○ **ME** ○ **YOU**   ○ **ME** ○ **YOU**

You don't like to prolong or sugarcoat things. Your bluntness is your biggest strength *and* your biggest weakness in relationships. This person is not a fan of tedious discussions and works best with someone who's equally frank and a little thick-skinned.

You crave quality time with your partner and prefer doing simple things that allow you the chance to be really close and talk. If this is the person you're with, plan a date that's all about being one-on-one. Some ideas: staying in bed all day or strolling through a museum.

MAKE HER FEEL SEXY NAKED

Together, check out these suggestions from Cosmo— and then see which ones will make your relationship steamier!

One way to make a woman feel great about how she looks sans clothing is to give little compliments at random times such as:

1. **"Are you working out more? You've been looking even hotter than usual."**

2. **"Man, you look incredible in that bra."**

3. **"You have no idea how often I think about how lucky I am to be with a girl with a body like yours."**

4. **"You look so good when you're on top of me."**

5. **"Sometimes I catch other guys checking you out as you walk by. I know I should be mad, but I can't really blame them."**

6. **"Please bend over again, your ass looks *sooo* good when you do that."**

7. **"Do you know how perfect your breasts are? They're the best I've ever seen."**

Of the compliments above, note your three favorites:

#_____ **HERE'S WHY**_____

_____

_____

#_____ **HERE'S WHY**_____

_____

_____

#_____ **HERE'S WHY**_____

_____

And here's one I didn't think of:

_____

_____

_____

_____

_____

_____

"THE TALK": WHEN HE WANTS IT MORE THAN YOU DO

If you don't seem as interested in sex as you usually do, he shouldn't take it personally. There are many reasons a woman may not be in the mood…and none of them have to do with you not being into him. Here are some of the most common explanations and some ways to overcome them—when you're done filling everything out, show your guy your answers.

REASON #1: YOU'VE BEEN TOGETHER FOR A WHILE

You know how when you were first dating, you were practically animals, ready to rip each other's clothes off at any given moment? That's because in the early stages, you probably didn't see each other that regularly, so it was like you had to get it on every time you were together. But now that you have a steady pattern of being together, you might not feel the need to always go at it. You know he'll be around later, so you're not as frantic about getting naked right this second. Feeding into this is the fact that guys can get a bit lazy! In the beginning, your man felt like he really had to woo you to get you into the sack. But now that you're a sure thing, he's stopped doing some of that stuff.

○ **THIS SOUNDS LIKE WHAT'S HAPPENING IN OUR RELATIONSHIP**

○ **THIS DOESN'T SOUND LIKE WHAT'S HAPPENING IN OUR RELATIONSHIP**

HOW TO PROCEED:

You can try initiating more spontaneous sex and start feeling that thrill from when you first met. And if he starts doing some of those little moves that have fallen by the wayside, it'll get you in the mood. Here are some Cosmo-approved ways for him to rekindle that spark—mark the ones you'd dig:

Surprise her with a kiss when she's doing something routine, like drying her hair.

○ I'D LIKE THIS   ○ MMM, I'LL PASS

Pause your favorite show and jump her. (Just don't make her spill her wine!)

○ I'D LIKE THIS   ○ MMM, I'LL PASS

After ordering food to be delivered, pin her to the couch and see if you can do it before the food arrives.

○ I'D LIKE THIS   ○ MMM, I'LL PASS

Here are some other ideas you've come up with together:

_____

_____

_____

REASON #2: YOU'RE STRESSED OUT

When you have a lot on your plate at work or are dealing with serious family issues, your first thought isn't hitting the sack.

○ THIS SOUNDS LIKE WHAT'S HAPPENING IN OUR RELATIONSHIP

○ THIS DOESN'T SOUND LIKE WHAT'S HAPPENING IN OUR RELATIONSHIP

HOW TO PROCEED:

If he senses that something is eating at you, now's not the time to push for action. Instead, he should try to ease the pressure on you in some creative ways. You never know—showing that he cares and being understanding just may be arousing. Check the options below that you're into.

Being affectionate definitely helps me de-stress. I'd love it if you:

○ CUDDLED WITH ME ON THE COUCH

○ GAVE ME A MASSAGE

○ TOOK A BATH OR SHOWER WITH ME

Here's another idea of my own:

_____

_____

_____

REASON #3: YOUR SEX DRIVE IS LOWER THAN HIS
Libido is biological to some degree, and it just may be that yours don't match up. The good news is that a person's sex drive ebbs and flows over the course of a lifetime, so if they aren't equal now, they might sync up at some point. Medical conditions and prescriptions can also cause a drop in sex drive. Depression, certain types of birth control, and even antibiotics can decrease libido. So it's never a bad idea to remind each other to go to the doctor for a physical to make sure everything's all right.

○ **I THINK THIS MAY BE THE CASE WITH ME,
AND I'D BE WILLING TO GET HELP**

○ **THIS IS DEFINITELY NOT THE CASE WITH ME**

Of all three reasons, I think #_____applies to me the most. And that's

because_____

_____

_____

Or, I don't think any of the reasons really apply to me. When I'm not as into

sex as you are, it's because_____

_____

_____

_____

_____

_____

CHAPTER 2

K-I-S-S-I-N-G

HOW SHE LIKES TO BE KISSED

Most women love kissing and want to do it as often as possible. Did you know that a man's saliva carries testosterone, and when he transfers that to you, it actually increases your sex drive? The trick is to start softly and then get more aggressive. Cosmo rounded up these tips—read them together and mark how you feel about each one! He'll be enlightened.

FOR HER

THE WARM-UP

Your man warms you up before launching into full-throttle passion. "Part of what excites her is the slow, steady build of a kiss," says Bloom. "So it's much more erotic to begin with light smooches."

○ **I LIKE LIGHT SMOOCHES**

○ **I'M NOT A FAN OF LIGHT SMOOCHES**

THE PECKER

This is when your guy gives you little pecks all over your cheeks and neck—totally avoiding your mouth. Once he can sense you aching for lip-on-lip action, he traces the outline of your mouth with his tongue.

○ **SOUNDS HOT**

○ **SOUNDS SILLY; I'D RATHER YOU JUST FOCUS ON MY MOUTH ALL THE TIME**

THE NO TONGUE

Your guy moves on to open-mouth kissing but keeps the anticipation building by not using his tongue.

○ **I LOVE IT WHEN YOU WITHHOLD TONGUE ACTION**

○ **I'D MISS YOUR TONGUE. GIVE IT TO ME, PLEASE!**

THE HARD PRESS

After starting with a soft French kiss, he varies the intensity of his lip-locks, like by pressing his lips against yours—hard.

○ **I LOVE HARD LIP PRESSES**

○ **I PREFER SOFT FRENCH KISSES ALWAYS**

THE CIRCLE

Here's where he swirls his tongue around yours in a circular motion—this creates a new sensation that's surprising and fun.

○ **I LIKE IT WHEN YOU SWIRL YOUR TONGUE AROUND MINE**

○ **I THINK THIS SOUNDS WEIRD AND WOULD PREFER IF YOU DIDN'T DO IT**

CROWDSOURCING SOME KISSING TECHNIQUES

Cosmo asked women how they like to be kissed. Mark if you agree or disagree with these, and have your guy read your answers!

THE NECK NOOKY **"One thing that sends me over the edge is when a guy gently grabs the hair at the back of my neck and lightly pulls it to angle my face up to his before swooping in for a lip-lock."** *—Sarah, 26*

○ I AGREE   ○ I DISAGREE

HERE'S WHY:

_____

_____

THE DEEP STARE **"I prefer romantic kisses, so when a man looks deeply into my eyes beforehand, it makes the entire experience feel more sensual."** *—Kristen, 24*

○ I AGREE   ○ I DISAGREE

HERE'S WHY:

_____

_____

THE WALL PRESS "I love when a guy presses me up against a wall while laying one on me. It makes it feel even more intense." —Dina, 32

◯ I AGREE ◯ I DISAGREE

HERE'S WHY:

_____

_____

THE GRAB "It's pretty simple: Reach down and grab my ass while your mouth is on mine. It is animalistic and revs me up." —Jenn, 30

◯ I AGREE ◯ I DISAGREE

HERE'S WHY:

_____

_____

THE TALKER "When a guy talks to me in between kisses, it can make things so much hotter. All he has to do is pull back every once in a while and tell me how much he likes me." —Jessie, 23

◯ I AGREE ◯ I DISAGREE

HERE'S WHY:

_____

_____

CHAPTER 3

HER BIGGEST TURN-ONS

LET'S START FROM THE TOP: HER BREASTS

Here are 15 Cosmo-endorsed boob moves for sexy foreplay, in no particular order. Each of you should rank them in order of which ones you'd like to try the most. If you rank any of them equally, those "win." Then battle it out to see which ones you'll try!

1. Lightly run your fingertips in circles, starting on the outer edge of her breasts and zeroing in until you reach the areolae.
2. Use your tongue. Take one of her nipples gently between your teeth, then rub your tongue back and forth over it.

3. Leave her bra on. Run your hands over it—the lace has a slightly rough texture that feels great against the skin.

4. When you're lounging together on the couch watching TV, put your hand inside her bra and lightly scratch her breasts with your fingertips.

5. Apply lotion, and treat her girls to a sensual massage. Using a circular motion and medium pressure, rub from the base of the boobs up along the outer edges, stopping just below the armpits. Then place your hands on her breastbone and work your way across the center of her chest, out toward the sides of her body.

6. Trace a figure eight around both nipples while giving her a deep, steamy kiss.

7. Get creative with whatever's around the house—trail a silk scarf, leather glove, or velour blanket over her breasts. Experiment with different textures to see what feels best against the sensitive skin.

8. Slather her twins with edible lotion, like Victoria's Secret Berry Passion, then enjoy that treat by running your tongue over them.

9. Unhook her bra without using your hands—c'mon, we dare you!

10. Grab a vibrator and run it back and forth across her breasts and nipples for an added jolt of pleasure. (For more sexy ways to use a vibrator, turn to page 91.)

11. Ask her to go crazy with massage oil on your back and use her breasts to give you a sensual rubdown.

12. During foreplay, pop a mint and then lick her nipples.

13. Stand in front of the bathroom mirror and cup her breasts from behind as you kiss her neck.

14. Have her squirt some lotion on your chest and stomach and then rub it in using nothing by her bare breasts.

15. Place an ice cube between her breasts and run it back and forth so that her skin feels cool and wet, then have her guide your penis between them for a hands-free massage.

Now let's each rank our favorites:

<table>
<tr><td>———— FOR HIM ————</td><td>———— FOR HER ————</td></tr>
<tr><td>1. _____</td><td>1. _____</td></tr>
<tr><td>2. _____</td><td>2. _____</td></tr>
<tr><td>3. _____</td><td>3. _____</td></tr>
<tr><td>4. _____</td><td>4. _____</td></tr>
<tr><td>5. _____</td><td>5. _____</td></tr>
<tr><td>6. _____</td><td>6. _____</td></tr>
<tr><td>7. _____</td><td>7. _____</td></tr>
<tr><td>8. _____</td><td>8. _____</td></tr>
<tr><td>9. _____</td><td>9. _____</td></tr>
<tr><td>10. _____</td><td>10. _____</td></tr>
<tr><td>11. _____</td><td>11. _____</td></tr>
<tr><td>12. _____</td><td>12. _____</td></tr>
<tr><td>13. _____</td><td>13. _____</td></tr>
<tr><td>14. _____</td><td>14. _____</td></tr>
<tr><td>15. _____</td><td>15. _____</td></tr>
</table>

———————————— FOR HER ————————————

Here are a few other ways to play with my breasts to turn up the heat:

_____

_____

_____

GAME TIME!

Cosmo asked a bunch of real women what they love and hate about foreplay. Read these with your guy, share how you feel about them, and expect some upgrades the next time you're getting busy.

FIRST UP: "I LOVE IT WHEN..."

THE ROUGH STUFF
"Men shouldn't be afraid to get a little rough during foreplay. Nothing turns me on more than when a guy uses his teeth to lightly graze my nipples, moves me where he wants me to be, or firmly grabs my ass as we kiss." —*Sara, 24*

◯ I AGREE   ◯ I DISAGREE

HERE'S WHY:

_____

_____

_____

THE TRAIL BLAZER
"When a guy kisses a trail from my breasts to my belly button, I go crazy. It's sensual, romantic, and hot." —*Deb, 26*

◯ I AGREE   ◯ I DISAGREE

HERE'S WHY:

_____

_____

THE SILLY WILLY
"I like it when a guy doesn't take himself too seriously in the bedroom. If he turns on fun, upbeat music, it excites me because I know he's looking for a good time and isn't going to be up-tight in bed."
—*Sue, 30*

○ I AGREE   ○ I DISAGREE

HERE'S WHY:

_____

_____

_____

UNDRESS TO IMPRESS
"There's some-thing erotic about a man undressing me—taking off my clothes one item at a time, stopping to kiss me deeply every once in a while."
—*Lauren, 25*

○ I AGREE   ○ I DISAGREE

HERE'S WHY:

_____

_____

_____

THE NECK NIBBLE

"I could almost orgasm from neck kissing alone. Seriously, the way to get me really wet is to spend a lot of time kissing there. Then switch it up and lick a trail from the bottom of my ear to my collarbone and back. It feels incredibly sensual, and that is such a sensitive spot that makes me tingle all over."

—Carrie, 28

○ I AGREE   ○ I DISAGREE

HERE'S WHY:

_____

_____

_____

My favorite moves from the above, ranked from 1 to 5, with 1 being the best:

_____ **The Rough Stuff**

_____ **The Trail Blazer**

_____ **The Silly Willy**

_____ **Undress to Impress**

_____ **The Neck Nibble**

NOW LET'S SWITCH IT UP:

THE DOWNTOWN DIEHARD "A lot of guys can go down on a girl and then expect that she can have sex right away. I love oral, but need my other body parts—like my boobs and lips—engaged too." —*Dina, 31*

○ I AGREE   ○ I DISAGREE

HERE'S WHY:

_____

_____

_____

THE LICKER "Yes, ears are sensitive and an erogenous zone, so please kiss near them or nibble on them. But when a guy licks inside my ear, it gives me the heebie-jeebies!" —*Natalie, 22*

○ I AGREE   ○ I DISAGREE

HERE'S WHY:

_____

_____

_____

TWIST AND SHOUT "Nipple twisting is not hot. They aren't dials that you can turn. Lick them, bite them, suck them . . . but do not twist!" —Kate, 25

◯ I AGREE　　◯ I DISAGREE

HERE'S WHY:

_____

_____

_____

THE GREAT EXPECTATION "I can't stand it when a guy gives me oral only because he wants it in return. I'm more than happy to give you a blow job, but when I feel like you're heading south just for that reason, it pisses me off." —Tasha, 34

◯ I AGREE　　◯ I DISAGREE

HERE'S WHY:

_____

_____

_____

THE ROUTINE ROMP

"I once dated a guy who would use the same routine every time we had sex: He'd spend a few minutes kissing me, fondle my breasts for another three minutes, then touch me down below for a bit. It was always the same and got boring really quickly."

—Ann, 29

○ I AGREE   ○ I DISAGREE

HERE'S WHY:

_____

_____

_____

My top five least favorite moves, ranked from 1 to 5, with 1 being the worst:

_____The Downtown Diehard

_____The Licker

_____Twist and Shout

_____The Great Expectation

_____The Routine Romp

FOREPLAY RULES EVERY MAN SHOULD FOLLOW

On average, it takes a woman 10 to 20 minutes to become completely aroused. So start by telling her how sexy she is (she'll never get sick of hearing that) and how good you want to make her feel. Then try these:

FOLLOW THIS MAKE-HER-MOAN MAP

Starting at her neck, teasingly graze her skin with your lips, like you were going to kiss her but changed your mind. Then nip and suck on her earlobe. Stand behind her and run your fingers up and down her arms. Hold her hair to one side and kiss all along her shoulders. Massage the base of her neck, then move to the front to stroke her breasts. Run your lips over her breasts, inner thighs, pelvis, and the curve above her hip.

GIVE HER A HAND

The clitoris plays a vital role in her arousal and, eventually, her orgasm. But she has a lot of other territory that will respond to your touch. When she shivers, sighs, or leans into your touch, you know you've hit a hot spot! Some suggestions: Trace your fingertips around the edges of her undies. Gently massage her upper inner thighs. When she's noticeably steamed up (her body writhing before you is a hint), lightly stroke her clitoris. With your index, middle, and ring fingers together (remember the Boy Scout salute?), press the flat part of your fingers—not the tips— against her vulva and rub it like you'd massage a muscle—gently but firmly in a circle. If you're not sure about pressure level, err on the side of too soft. If she presses against you or seems anxious for more, increase your pressure.

GIVE SOME LIP SERVICE

Your tongue can provide a unique (and ecstasy-producing) sensation to her vagina. When you're taking off her underwear, go through the layers, touching and licking over her undies, dampening them, and then inching them off. Forget about patenting some complicated tongue twister—that's one of the biggest mistakes a guy can make. A good, basic oral sex technique is tracing a figure eight with your tongue. The reason it works: Instead of hitting the same spots repeatedly, you stimulate the whole area. To get a feel for the other things she likes, flick your tongue lightly around the sides and top of her vulva. Draw circles around it with the tip of your tongue. Kiss her there the same way you would her mouth and she'll see stars.

Here's a cheat sheet that tells you what foreplay moves will get her hot—or not! Have her mark her answer for each.

WHEN YOU'RE: Touching her inner thighs

PRETEND YOU'RE: Working clay. It gets blood pumping through that region, priming her for sex.

○ I LIKE THE IDEA OF THIS   ○ THIS SOUNDS STRANGE

WHEN YOU'RE: Nipping at the base of her neck

PRETEND YOU'RE: Lightly taking sesame seeds off a bun with your teeth

○ SOUNDS DELICIOUS   ○ SOUNDS WEIRD

WHEN YOU'RE: Slipping off her clothes and underwear

PRETEND YOU'RE: Peeling fruit. Do it slowly and carefully.

○ OH, YEAH!   ○ ACTUALLY, I'M OKAY WITH
                      YOU RIPPING MY CLOTHES OFF

WHEN YOU'RE: Going south of the border

PRETEND YOU'RE: Licking a stamp, only muuuch slower

○ THIS SOUNDS AWESOME   ○ I'D PREFER YOU GO SLOW
                                SOMETIMES AND FAST AT
                                OTHER TIMES. MIX IT UP.

ORAL REPORT!

Cosmo rounded up the top oral moves sure to wow most women. Can you guess which move is her favorite? (Have her mark her fave at the bottom.)

FOR HIM

THE WINDSHIELD WIPER

Point your tongue and move it in an arc up and over her clitoris. Keep repeating until she's squirming with desire.

THE SNAKE

Place your mouth right over the opening of her vagina. Then stick out your tongue and flick it in and out of her, like a snake. The entrance of her V zone is where most of the nerves are, so it'll feel extra good.

THE SENSUAL SUCK

Stick out your lips (as if you were going to give her a peck), place them around her clitoris, and gently suck. Instead of providing direct stimulation, this puts heavenly pressure on that sexy spot.

THE KITTY KAT

Start at the bottom of her vagina and lick up to her clitoris and then back down—like a cat lapping up milk.

THE ONE-TWO PUNCH

While using your tongue to lavishly lick her clitoris, slip two fingers inside her and move them in and out. Start by moving your tongue and fingers slowly and keep increasing the speed. This combo of clitoral and vaginal stimulation feels great.

THE CRAZY 8

If all else fails, this should take her over the edge: Point your tongue and, starting above her clitoris, move it in a figure-eight pattern, going around the edges of the clit to give her indirect but intense stimulation.

Here's how I'd rank the above from 1 to 6, with 1 being my absolute favorite:

_____ **The Windshield Wiper**   _____ **The Snake**

_____ **The Sensual Suck**   _____ **The Kitty Kat**

_____ **The One-Two Punch**   _____ **The Crazy 8**

I picked _____ **as my top choice because**

_____

_____

_____

_____

_____

_____

_____

_____

_____

_____

_____

LET'S TALK ABOUT SEX, BABY

CHAPTER 4

CAUGHT IN THE ACT

HER FAVORITE POSITIONS

*And now, the chapter you've been waiting for:
a tantalizing guide of passion poses and steamy
sexcapades that you can peruse together...
and then pursue together.*

If you're like most people, you have certain positions in your sexual
repertoire that you return to again and again because they're most likely
to get you to maximum pleasure. But repeatedly falling back on the same
positions can leave you in an erotic rut. In this chapter, you'll discover the
positions that are most guaranteed to give her an orgasm (which is a win
for him, too!), the positions that will make you feel emotionally—not just
physically—closer as a couple, the best sex position for every mood, and
the positions that'll turn your sex life on its head, spicing things up in ways
neither of you never imagined. Ready to get started?

THE G-SPOT JIGGY

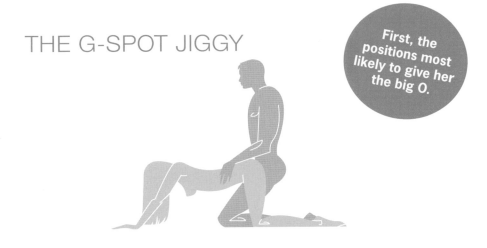

First, the positions most likely to give her the big O.

FOR HIM

HOW YOU'LL DO THIS:

Have her get down on all fours while you kneel behind her, and then it's on you to literally just plunge inside her. (Feel free to grab her butt for balance!) Thrust far enough inside her so that your testicles hit her body. This will feel *amazing* for her—trust us.

FOR HER

Aside from the fact that I can easily orgasm, I love this position because _____

_____

_____

And I'd love it even more if you _____

_____

_____

_____

HOT HULA

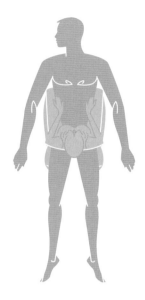

HOW YOU'LL DO THIS:

Lie on your back with a pillow propped under your head. Then, have her face you and lower herself onto your penis, putting her hands and knees on either side of you. Enter her deeply and swivel your hips from side to side, potentially all around—and have her do the same.

FOR HER

Aside from the fact that I can easily orgasm, I love this position because _____

_____

_____

And I'd love it even more if you _____

_____

_____

_____

_____

THE PASSION PYTHON

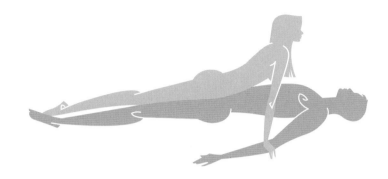

FOR HIM

HOW YOU'LL DO THIS:

Lie flat on your back, and have her straddle you and lower herself onto your penis. Then she should stretch out slowly, so she's lying straight on top of you, aligned limb to limb. Holding each other's hands, extend your arms out to your sides as she lifts her torso. Keep your feet flexed so she can push against them with her toes for leverage.

FOR HER

Aside from the fact that I can easily orgasm, I love this position because _____

_____

_____

And I'd love it even more if you _____

_____

_____

_____

STANDING TIGER, CROUCHING DRAGON

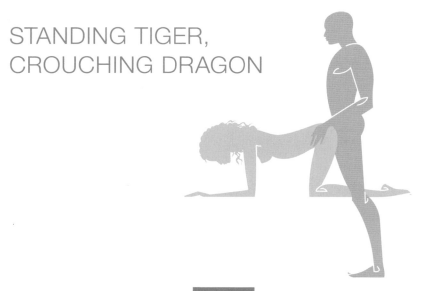

HOW YOU'LL DO THIS:

Have her get down on all fours, with her knees at the edge of the bed, and stand behind her, feet hip-width apart. Then spread your legs on either side of hers and thrust. Have her keep her knees together as you thrust.

FOR HER

Aside from the fact that I can easily orgasm, I love this position because _____

_____

_____

And I'd love it even more if you _____

_____

_____

_____

_____

THE HOT SEAT

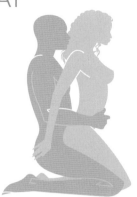

FOR HIM

HOW YOU'LL DO THIS:

Kneel behind her, leaning slightly backward. Then have her kneel in front of you, with her back toward you and legs between yours. Your bodies should be squeezed together tightly. Wrap your arms around her waist and, once you're inside her, swivel your hips in a circular motion so you're in tandem. Stop for a break when you get too worked up or tired.

FOR HER

Aside from the fact that I can easily orgasm, I love this position because _____

_____

_____

And I'd love it even more if you _____

_____

_____

_____

GET DOWN ON IT

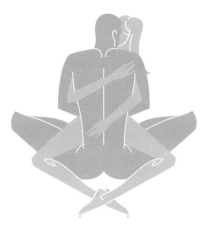

FOR HER

HOW YOU'LL DO THIS:

First, get into the traditional Lotus position, with your legs crossed and each of your heels atop the opposite knee. Then face your guy, sit in his lap, and mount him, with your legs wrapped snugly around his waist. Embrace each other (awww) and kiss so that as you exhale, he inhales, and vice versa. Then, he mirrors your movements: As he breathes in, rock your pelvis back and tighten your vagina; as he exhales, rock your pelvis forward and release.

Aside from the fact that I can easily orgasm, I love this position because _____

_____

_____

And I'd love it even more if you _____

_____

_____

_____

_____

TORRID TUG-OF-WAR

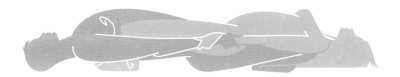

HOW YOU'LL DO THIS:

Sit cross-legged on the floor or the bed and straddle him. Lower yourself onto his penis and have him wrap his legs around your back. As you're sitting face-to-face, grab each other's elbows and then lean back against each other's weight—kind of like tug-of-war. Hold as still as possible so you can really concentrate on your connection.

Aside from the fact that I can easily orgasm, I love this position because _____

_____

_____

And I'd love it even more if you _____

_____

_____

_____

_____

SAUCY SPOONS

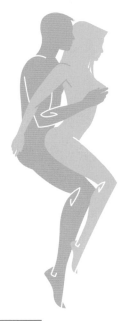

FOR HER

HOW YOU'LL DO THIS:

Have him lie on his side behind you so you're both facing the same direction. Push your butt toward him as he enters you. Have him bring his hand around and touch your clitoris—it'll be awesome—and then alternate between there and your breasts.

Aside from the fact that I can easily orgasm, I love this position because _____

_____

_____

And I'd love it even more if you _____

_____

_____

_____

_____

THE HANG TEN

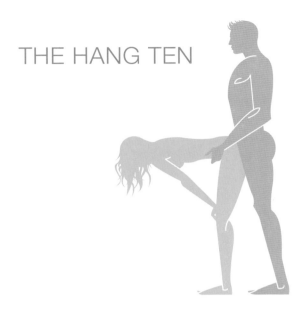

HOW YOU'LL DO THIS:

First, bend forward with your legs spread, back straight, and hands resting on your knees for balance. Then it's on your guy to enter you from behind, pulling himself as close to you as possible while holding your torso for support. Have him bring you even closer until your bodies come into full contact. He can lean slightly over you to gain pumping power.

Aside from the fact that I can easily orgasm, I love this position because _____

_____

_____

And I'd love it even more if you _____

_____

_____

_____

TIME BOMB

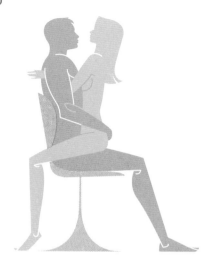

FOR HER

HOW YOU'LL DO THIS:

Have him sit in a low chair with his legs relaxed. Face him and straddle him with your feet on the floor, slowly lowering yourself onto him. He should enter you with just the tip of his penis at first; then lower yourself inch by inch until you get full entry.

Aside from the fact that I can easily orgasm, I love this position because _____

_____

_____

And I'd love it even more if you _____

_____

_____

_____

_____

NOW AND ZEN

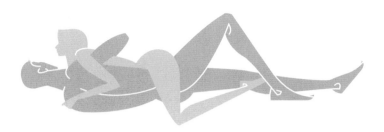

HOW YOU'LL DO THIS:

When you're both on the brink of the big O, take a break and roll onto your sides, face-to-face (if possible, have him stay inside you the entire time). Then, intertwine your legs, being sure to keep his chest pressed against yours the whole time. This will slowly build you back up so your orgasms are more incredible than ever!

Aside from the fact that I can easily orgasm, I love this position because _____

_____

_____

And I'd love it even more if you _____

_____

_____

_____

4 WAYS TO GET SCHMOOPY DURING SEX

Cosmo asked sexologist Joy Davidson, PhD, for tips on how to have super-intimate sex. Check them out, answer the questions below individually, and then share with each other so you know how the other feels about these romantic moments. (Or read 'em aloud and try to guess each other's answers!)

UNDRESS EACH OTHER

Rather than each ripping off your own clothes, do it for each other. "It forces you to slow down and lets her know she is the center of your attention," says Davidson. "Plus, it revs her up, because you end up naturally stroking her as the fabric slides along her skin."

How hot do *you* think this is?
- ○ SO HOT
- ○ SORTA HOT
- ○ NOT HOT

How hot does *he* think this is?
- ○ SO HOT
- ○ SORTA HOT
- ○ NOT HOT

PRESS AGAINST HER

When you're about to climax, have him hold his body tightly against yours. If you're in missionary, have him wrap his arms around your back and hug you. Or if you're on top, have him pull your shoulders down to him so that you're chest to chest. "Doing this reminds her you're in this together," says Davidson.

How hot do *you* think this is?
- ○ SO HOT
- ○ SORTA HOT
- ○ NOT HOT

How hot does *he* think this is?
- ○ SO HOT
- ○ SORTA HOT
- ○ NOT HOT

MAKE EYE CONTACT

Holding each other's gaze is a really powerful way to feel bonded. During sex, have him angle his head slightly to the right so that the left side of his face is aligned with the left side of yours, and look each other in the eye. Just don't get too intense or it'll seem like you're trying to bore holes through each other's skull.

How hot do *you* think this is?
- ◯ SO HOT
- ◯ SORTA HOT
- ◯ NOT HOT

How hot does *he* think this is?
- ◯ SO HOT
- ◯ SORTA HOT
- ◯ NOT HOT

BE STILL FOR A MOMENT

While he's on top, stay completely motionless for a few seconds. Then ask him to whisper something sexy in your ear. It builds the anticipation so that when you start moving again, it feels that much more intense and incredible.

How hot do *you* think this is?
- ◯ SO HOT
- ◯ SORTA HOT
- ◯ NOT HOT

How hot does *he* think this is?
- ◯ SO HOT
- ◯ SORTA HOT
- ◯ NOT HOT

Now, each rank your favorite moves from 1 to 4, with 1 being your favorite:

1: _____
2: _____
3: _____
4: _____

1: _____
2: _____
3: _____
4: _____

(Hopefully, you had similar answers!)

TRIED & THRUSTED

Here are three of the most common types of thrusting. Note which thrust position is your favorite below, show your guy—and then, um, have him act accordingly!

THE CORKSCREW

Think about how you twist a screw in. When your guy does the same motion with his penis, it'll rock your world. There is a reason they call it screwing, after all. He should go as deep as possible inside you and then rotate his hips in a big circle. He'll hit parts of your vaginal walls that straight in-and-out thrusting misses, and his pelvis will grind against your clitoris for double pleasure.

THE QUICK AND SHALLOW

Since the first three inches of your vagina is where the most nerves are, you'll feel his penis there. So if he keeps his thrusting shallow, it'll maximize the feel-good sensations. And if he does it quickly, it'll create more friction, adding to both of your pleasure.

THE JACKHAMMER

Sometimes guys get carried away and start pounding a bit too hard and fast. Even though you see this move in porn all the time, it doesn't really feel good. However, quick, forceful thrusts can feel great when combined with slower, softer moves. It's all about knowing what you want in the moment. Guys: If you get the vibe she's not feeling it ("ouch" is a good clue), slow down to a more leisurely pace.

Here are my favorite thrusting techniques, in order from most favorite to least favorite:

1. _____

2. _____

3. _____

When I'm feeling schmoopy, I like_____best.

When I'm feeling wild and crazy, I like_____best.

When it's late after a party, I like it when you do _____

When we first wake up, _____
is my favorite thrusting technique of yours.

SEX MOVES TO MATCH EVERY MOOD

Sometimes insane, contortionist, bend-over-backward-and-balance-on-one-hand sex isn't necessarily what either of you is craving. Luckily, Cosmo has a sex move for 14 varying emotional states. Take a look and see which ones you like best—then remember them the next time you're in that kind of mood.

CUDDLY

Lie with your head on his chest and trace cute little messages across his torso ("So happy," "You're hot," etc.). Then let him reciprocate by writing his own love note across your back.

How hot do *you* think this is?
- ○ SO HOT
- ○ SORTA HOT
- ○ NOT HOT

How hot does *he* think this is?
- ○ SO HOT
- ○ SORTA HOT
- ○ NOT HOT

SEXY/BEAUTIFUL

Your hair is behaving brilliantly, and you're owning your skinny jeans: Now is the time to show off the goods. Straddle him while he's lying face-up on the bed, and lean back so your elbows are resting behind you. He can thrust up while getting an eyeful of your rocking bod.

How hot do *you* think this is?
- ⃝ SO HOT
- ⃝ SORTA HOT
- ⃝ NOT HOT

How hot does *he* think this is?
- ⃝ SO HOT
- ⃝ SORTA HOT
- ⃝ NOT HOT

SHY

This is the perfect time to employ half-dressed sex: Keep your minidress on, push your undies aside, and don't let him take off his pants all the way—it'll feel urgent and charged, without putting you on full display.

How hot do *you* think this is?
- ⃝ SO HOT
- ⃝ SORTA HOT
- ⃝ NOT HOT

How hot does *he* think this is?
- ⃝ SO HOT
- ⃝ SORTA HOT
- ⃝ NOT HOT

NAUGHTY

Go commando on a date while he's driving or while you're sitting in the movie theater, slyly slip his hand underneath your skirt, and give him a saucy little smile. He'll know that when you get home later, it's on.

How hot do *you* think this is?
- ⃝ SO HOT
- ⃝ SORTA HOT
- ⃝ NOT HOT

How hot does *he* think this is?
- ⃝ SO HOT
- ⃝ SORTA HOT
- ⃝ NOT HOT

CRAZY

Doggie-style sex—in front of a window!—taps into your wild, exhibitionist side. You'll literally steam things up.

How hot do *you* think this is?
- ○ SO HOT
- ○ SORTA HOT
- ○ NOT HOT

How hot does *he* think this is?
- ○ SO HOT
- ○ SORTA HOT
- ○ NOT HOT

VOYEURISTIC

Ask him to touch himself while you watch. It's hot to see your guy completely lose control while you maintain it. Plus—learning opportunity!

How hot do *you* think this is?
- ○ SO HOT
- ○ SORTA HOT
- ○ NOT HOT

How hot does *he* think this is?
- ○ SO HOT
- ○ SORTA HOT
- ○ NOT HOT

LAZY

Have a pizza picnic party in bed. No TV allowed: Put on a sexy playlist, and sit across from each other like you would at a restaurant. Serve the pizza on plates, pour some wine, and don't be afraid to get messy.

How hot do *you* think this is?
- ○ SO HOT
- ○ SORTA HOT
- ○ NOT HOT

How hot does *he* think this is?
- ○ SO HOT
- ○ SORTA HOT
- ○ NOT HOT

EXPERIMENTAL

Hot-cold play is when you alternate sensations to build tension, because you don't know which you're going to experience next. Take turns blindfolding each other and teasing sensitive spots like the neck, nipples, and inner thighs with ice cubes and your warm breath.

How hot do *you* think this is?
- ○ SO HOT
- ○ SORTA HOT
- ○ NOT HOT

How hot does *he* think this is?
- ○ SO HOT
- ○ SORTA HOT
- ○ NOT HOT

ROMANTIC

Dim the lights and trade backrubs. Massages release the bonding hormone oxytocin, so you'll feel even more connected to each other.

How hot do *you* think this is?
- ○ SO HOT
- ○ SORTA HOT
- ○ NOT HOT

How hot does *he* think this is?
- ○ SO HOT
- ○ SORTA HOT
- ○ NOT HOT

PLAYFUL

All that pushing and rubbing up against each other? Yes, play-wrestling can be super sexy and fun. Just be sure to hold the smackdown on an area with a soft surface—like your mattress or a fuzzy carpet.

How hot do *you* think this is?
- ○ SO HOT
- ○ SORTA HOT
- ○ NOT HOT

How hot does *he* think this is?
- ○ SO HOT
- ○ SORTA HOT
- ○ NOT HOT

TAKE-CHARGE

Climb on top of him and pin his wrists against the bed. Holding onto his arms gives you leverage so you can really go for it and adds to the you-in-control vibe. The diagonal angle also provides more contact between his pelvic bone and your clitoris, upping the orgasmic potential.

How hot do *you* think this is?
- ◯ SO HOT
- ◯ SORTA HOT
- ◯ NOT HOT

How hot does *he* think this is?
- ◯ SO HOT
- ◯ SORTA HOT
- ◯ NOT HOT

SUBMISSIVE

Have him bind your wrists behind your back with one of his ties before he goes down on you.

How hot do *you* think this is?
- ◯ SO HOT
- ◯ SORTA HOT
- ◯ NOT HOT

How hot does *he* think this is?
- ◯ SO HOT
- ◯ SORTA HOT
- ◯ NOT HOT

STRESSED

Orgasms are tension busters, so after a hard day at work, pull your guy close and whisper, "All I want is for you to make me come." (Hel-lo!)

How hot do *you* think this is?
- ◯ SO HOT
- ◯ SORTA HOT
- ◯ NOT HOT

How hot does *he* think this is?
- ◯ SO HOT
- ◯ SORTA HOT
- ◯ NOT HOT

KINKY

On nights when you want to let your freak flag fly, assume an alter ego. It's easier to get into character when you don't look like you, so meet him at the door wearing a wig and tell him, "Your girlfriend is working late tonight. I'm her evil twin." His night just got a lot more interesting. (For more ideas on role-playing, turn to page 81.)

How hot do *you* think this is?
- ◯ SO HOT
- ◯ SORTA HOT
- ◯ NOT HOT

How hot does *he* think this is?
- ◯ SO HOT
- ◯ SORTA HOT
- ◯ NOT HOT

──────── **FOR HER** ────────

Right now, I'm in the mood for _____

_____

These are the moves, if any, that I will probably never be in the mood for, and why:

_____

_____

_____

──────── **FOR HIM** ────────

Right now, I'm in the mood for _____

_____

These are the moves, if any, that I will probably never be in the mood for, and why:

_____

_____

_____

HOW TO KEEP IT HOT

Cosmo says that mixing up your sex routine brings mystery and adventure to your love life. Check out the seven sex styles and see how you feel about each one. Then have your man guess which ones may be out of your comfort zone—those are the styles to try the next time you feel like you're falling into a bit of a rut.

LIGHT-SPEED SEX

A quickie is kind of like an earthquake: It gets your adrenaline rushing, is over in a flash, and leaves you weak in the knees. In addition, a fast and furious romp really takes the edge off. When one of you is in a horny, hasty mood, don't bother fully undressing—just pull his penis out of the opening in his boxers and push your panties aside. All you need for successful speed sex is lube.

○ **I LOVE THIS**   ○ **THIS IS OUT OF MY COMFORT ZONE**

SHOWOFF SEX

You might think it'd be easier to give a speech in front of 500 people than to masturbate in front of your man, but taking that plunge is worth it—experts say that watching a woman pleasure herself is near the top of most men's fantasy wish lists. And it's not just a very personal peep show; it's a chance to teach him exactly how you like to be manhandled.

○ **I LOVE THIS**   ○ **THIS IS OUT OF MY COMFORT ZONE**

WILD-KINGDOM SEX

It's the raw, primal, grunting kind of sex that wakes the neighbors, and scares house pets. Any animalistic sex session starts, fittingly, on all fours. Grab his hands and wrap them around your waist—a cue that you want him to hold on and thrust—and he'll answer your call of the wild. And keep your neck down—it'll help you loosen up all the way down your spine so you can move your tush with gusto.

○ **I LOVE THIS**   ○ **THIS IS OUT OF MY COMFORT ZONE**

SURRENDER SEX

Men are conquest-loving creatures, which is why they get so hot when you let them take over. During foreplay, let your legs fall open and hold the headboard or pillows above you so your whole body is exposed to him. Then invite him to slide on top of you. Meet his thrusts halfway by rocking your pelvis upward against his and lifting your legs in the air with your feet spread far apart. This gives him room to maneuver his body and alternate between deep thrusting and short pumping. Then drape your legs over his shoulders so he can grab your ankles and position them where he wants them.

◯ I LOVE THIS   ◯ THIS IS OUT OF MY COMFORT ZONE

FEMALE-DOMINATION SEX

If he's been doing all the pouncing and pawing lately, take the reins. But it has to be authentic and not staged, so wait until you're really randy, straddle him, and say, "I'd love to be in charge tonight." Then gently grab his penis and rub it around your clitoris as if he were your personal sex toy. Once you slip him in, pin his hands to the bed or tie him to the headboard with scarves while you grind against his lap in a circular motion.

◯ I LOVE THIS   ◯ THIS IS OUT OF MY COMFORT ZONE

COMFORT SEX

Sometimes all you want is the sexual equivalent of mac and cheese: It may not be exciting, but it makes you feel so good. "Making each other feel loved and cared for is the most powerful way to bring the psychological and physical elements of your relationship together," says marital-sex therapist Michael Seiler, PhD.

◯ I THINK WE HAVE ENOUGH COMFORT SEX

◯ I DON'T THINK WE HAVE ENOUGH COMFORT SEX

CHAPTER 5

OH, OH, OH, OH, OH, *OHHH*

THE BASICS

Below, we've listed the three most common types of orgasms. Take some, uh, pleasure in marking your favorite. Then have your guy take notes.

CLITORAL

This is the most common type for a woman to have. But don't think that just because it's the usual, it's less special. Trust us, it feels sooo good. To give her one: Stimulate her clitoris during sex—it's easy to do this in girl-on-top, since her love button will be right in front of you. The key is to start slowly, and then rub a little more aggressively.

This is my favorite kind of O. _____

Especially when _____

_____

_____

_____

G-SPOT

Women often describe this climax as deeper or more intense. To give her one: You have to stimulate the G-spot during sex. It's situated about 2 inches up on the front wall of the vagina. You can hit this spot with your finger to push her to her limit, or you can try it during sex in the missionary position. Just prop up her butt with a few pillows so her pelvis is at the right angle to let you hit the area.

This is my favorite kind of O. _____

Especially when _____

_____

_____

_____

_____

_____

BLENDED

The first two Os are damn good in their own right. Now imagine combining the forces of both for one phenomenal finale. Well, that's what a blended orgasm is. To give her one: Have her lie on her back on the edge of the bed, with her feet dangling over the side and a few pillows underneath her butt to raise her pelvis (this makes it easier for you to hit the G-spot). Stand between her legs and, once you're thrusting, start teasing her clitoris until she reaches an explosive climax.

This is my favorite kind of O. _____

Especially when _____

_____

_____

_____

_____

_____

THE BIOLOGY BEHIND
HER ORGASM

Sex researchers from the Kinsey Institute forked over information for this graph, which shows how orgasms work for women. Check out each stage so you know what you're experiencing. (Hint: When you know which phase she's in, you'll be able to tailor your moves more easily!)

FOR HIM

EXCITEMENT

As soon as you start touching her in a sexy way, she gets excited and her body shows physical signs of it: Her skin becomes flushed, her nipples harden, and she begin to get wet down there.

PLATEAU

Once she's aroused, she reaches a bit of a standstill . . . and if you don't make the right moves, she may never hit that ultimate goal. That's because her body has gotten used to whatever you were doing during the excitement phase and needs different kinds of stimulation to get hot enough to peak. It's important to switch up your moves and not stick with the same pattern of touching, licking, and thrusting.

ORGASM

When she climaxes, it often comes on suddenly and lasts for about 15 to 18 seconds. Her vaginal muscles will flex involuntarily, her feet may spasm, and she may develop a flush across her chest.

RESOLUTION

During this phase, her body is slowly returning to its normal state. Feel-good hormones like dopamine and oxytocin are racing through her veins, making her feel happy and relaxed.

IS SHE SATISFIED?

An alternative to asking her "Did you come?" is to look for the telltale signs.

IF SHE'S PHYSICALLY AMPED

In the immediate aftermath of a satisfying sack session, her breathing will be rapid then slowly start to resume to a normal rhythm. Another clue that you rocked her world: Her skin, especially around the neck and chest area, might be flushed.

O YES   O NO

IF SHE PRAISES YOU

Pay attention to those compliments. "'Great' sounds positive, but her one-word summary could mean that she wants more and isn't telling you," says Tracey Cox, author of *Superhotsex*. But don't get discouraged. Break the ice with some humor, then ask her what would really make her toes curl. If she wasn't turned on the first time, she can still become very sexual when you encourage her to ask for more.

O YES   O NO

IF SHE GETS UP TO DO STUFF

When a woman is sexually gratified, she'll usually crave contact via cuddling, talking, or wanting to go for round two, says Darcy Luadzers, PhD, author of *The Ten-Minute Sexual Solution*. "When she's dissatisfied, she'll detach, which could entail rolling over or getting out of bed." So if she bolts to the kitchen to make a snack, flip on the television, or text a friend, it's not good, buddy. (Sorry, but you want the straight truth, don't you?) "Busying herself means that those things were either on her mind during the act or she wasn't satisfied and this is how she's channeling her frustration," adds Cox.

O YES   O NO

SAY THIS TO HER RIGHT AFTER SEX

Even if you did show her a good time, your job's not done . . . yet. Here's what she'd love to hear.

FOR HIM

"THAT FELT INCREDIBLE." Why she needs to hear it: Women feel performance anxiety too, so she wants reassurance that she's good in bed. Compliments increase her confidence.

"YOUR BODY IS SO SEXY." Why she needs to hear it: Intercourse can cause a woman to feel vulnerable and exposed, so praising her amazing stomach, for example, will boost how she feels when she's naked.

"HOW ARE YOU DOING?" Why she needs to hear it: She feels more bonded to you after sex, so checking in with her feeds her need to connect.

"SO, UH, WHAT'S YOUR NAME AGAIN?" Why she needs to hear it: Because she wants sex to have some levity and this line lends that—as long as you truly *are* kidding!

FOR HER

Rank your favorite things to hear after sex from 1 to 4, with 1 being what you love to hear the most:

"That felt incredible."_____

"Your body is so sexy."_____

"How are you doing?"_____

"So, uh, what's your name again?"_____

Besides the ones mentioned above, this is something else I love to hear:

_____

_____

CHAPTER 6

RIDIN' SOLO

THE TRUTH ABOUT SELF-LOVE

FOR HIM

Solo sex is a tricky subject when it comes to women—studies show that 92 percent do it, but many don't feel comfortable talking about it. Here's some advice for guys: Try to get her to chat about it with you and even ask her to masturbate in front of you. She knows her body best and can get herself off quickly and easily. So if you're able to watch, you'll pick up invaluable info. "Tell your girlfriend or wife that you can think of nothing more arousing than watching her pleasure herself," says sex therapist Judith Seifer, PhD. "If she feels weird about it, say you'll help her out by touching her in other places." It may take her a while to feel okay about doing it in front of you, but if you occasionally mention how fired up it would get you, she might want to try it.

In the meantime, learn what women told *Cosmo* about their self-lovin' tactics. Fill out the questions below to see how you compare.

A SENSUAL MOOD

"I make touching myself an event. I put on lotion, light some candles, and turn on music. It makes me feel taken care of and extra sexy." *—Gabrielle, 24*

◯ **I DO THIS**   ◯ **I DON'T DO THIS**

WHY OR WHY NOT:

_____

_____

_____

A LITTLE WARM-UP

"I run my fingers from my belly button to my nipples over and over. Warming up the rest of my body before concentrating on my clitoris helps big time." *—Melanie, 34*

◯ **I DO THIS**   ◯ **I DON'T DO THIS**

WHY OR WHY NOT:

_____

_____

_____

NOT THE TYPICAL PLACE

"I like to picture myself in the bathtub. The warm water is relaxing and sensual." **—Erin, 26**

○ **I DO THIS**   ○ **I DON'T DO THIS**

WHY OR WHY NOT:

_____

_____

_____

SWITCHING UP THE MOVES

"I rub my clitoris slowly and then speed up. Then I pull back and do it again, more leisurely. I go back and forth until I finally finish." **—Diane, 31**

○ **I DO THIS**   ○ **I DON'T DO THIS**

WHY OR WHY NOT:

_____

_____

_____

ADDING GADGETS

"I use a vibrator on my clitoris to really rev me up. Then when I'm close, I'll stick a finger inside myself. That almost always makes me orgasm." —*Laney, 29*

○ I DO THIS   ○ I DON'T DO THIS

WHY OR WHY NOT:

_____

_____

_____

Now, rank these moves from 1 to 5, with 1 being your favorite:

_____ **A Sensual Mood**

_____ **A Little Warm-Up**

_____ **Not the Typical Place**

_____ **Switching Up the Moves**

_____ **Adding Gadgets**

Describe your go-to move and why you dig it:

_____

_____

_____

_____

How do you feel about masturbating in front of your partner?

○ **I HAVE NO PROBLEM DOING SO**

○ **I WOULD LIKE TO, BUT I KIND OF FEEL EMBARRASSED**

○ **I WOULD NEVER.**

If you're on the fence about masturbating in front of your guy, what can he do to make you feel at ease?

_____

_____

_____

_____

_____

_____

HOW ABOUT SOME SEXTRAS?

CHAPTER 7

DIRTY TALK

STARTING OUT

Uttering something naughty while you're in the act can really heighten the entire experience. "It makes a woman feel more desirable, and that contributes to her climaxing more easily," says Cosmo contributor Aline Zoldbrod, PhD, coauthor of Sex Talk. *But keep in mind that while you might get off on hearing phrases cribbed from porn (more on that in the next chapter), most women prefer things that aren't as porn-y.*

Check out what Zoldbrod recommends men do before launching into dirty talk with a woman—then comment on these tactics below so your guy knows what you like.

TEST HER OUTSIDE THE BEDROOM

Say something like, "I was at the gym, thinking about your hot ass." If she seems intrigued, it's okay to bust out the naughty talk between the sheets. If not, you may have to stick with moans of pleasure to communicate how you feel in the moment.

START OFF SMALL

Getting too raunchy too fast could backfire. Ease into it by telling her how aroused she makes you. It's flattering and helps to cement an image of herself as desirable and alluring.

BE SPECIFIC

Talk about how amazing her breasts look and how you love grasping her awesome butt. Detailed compliments let her know that you worship her body specifically.

TAKE IT UP A NOTCH

If she volleys back with something just as frisky or belts out some keep-it-coming moaning, then tell her that you love the way she tastes and smells.

Here, tell your guy which of the previous advice from Dr. Zolbrod applies most to you, and why:

_____

_____

_____

_____

_____

DIRTY TALK THAT DRIVES HIM WILD

Here's what Cosmo recommends a woman say to a man in bed. Read these quotes together to learn why they work, and mark which ones you'd like to hear most from her.

"WHAT DO YOU WANT ME TO DO TO YOU?"

Asking him what he needs from you proves you're open to changing things up. Also, if you're talking dirty for the first time with your guy, this phrase is a good way to ease into conversation and gauge how naughty he's ready to get.

Do you want to hear this?   ○ YES   ○ NO

"YOU'RE AN AMAZING KISSER."

Not only will this deepen intimacy during foreplay, but since guys are performance-oriented, positive feedback emboldens him, heightening his arousal.

Do you want to hear this?   ○ YES   ○ NO

"I WANT YOU."

Since the signs of female arousal are much more subtle than male arousal (you can *clearly* see when he's frisky), he's eager for any affirmation that you're hot for him.

Do you want to hear this?   ○ YES   ○ NO

"F--- ME HARDER."

Pushing yourself outside of your comfort zone with words like "tits," "pussy," or "f---" conveys that your boundaries are down and lust has taken over. You don't want to sound phony, so only drop an f-bomb if it feels right to you. And make sure your language matches your level of arousal, becoming more explicit the closer you get to orgasm.

Do you want to hear this?   ◯ **YES**   ◯ **NO**

"IT FEELS INCREDIBLE WHEN YOU PRESS YOUR PENIS AGAINST ME."

Many guys have insecurities about their magic wand's size, shape, or appearance. So letting him know you love his penis boosts his confidence and gets him hornier.

Do you want to hear this?   ◯ **YES**   ◯ **NO**

"PUT YOUR MOUTH ON MY BREASTS."

Giving him a sexy command à la Christian Grey shows that you're confident, in control, and want to build the action even more—all huge turn-ons. Any sultry demand works; try approaching it like Mad Libs ("I want to play with your _____ " or "Grab my _____ ").

Do you want to hear this?   ◯ **YES**   ◯ **NO**

"I LOVE THE WAY YOU FILL ME UP."

Entering you is one of the most pleasurable moments of sex for a guy, because when he's pushing through your vagina for the first time, he feels like he's having an, ahem, big impact on you. Describing the sensation you experience when he penetrates you draws attention to the fact that you notice how huge and hard he is.

Do you want to hear this?   ◯ **YES**   ◯ **NO**

DIRTY TALK DEAL MAKERS—AND BREAKERS

Cosmo asked real women for the top things they love to hear a guy say—and what totally turns them off. Rank them in order from 1 to 8, at the same time have your guy guess how you rank them, and then see how well he did. (No peeking!)

SO, WHAT DO YOU THINK SHE WANTS TO HEAR IN BED?

"You're *sooo* hot." _____   "Did you come yet?" _____

"Now that I've gone down on you…" _____   "I love going down on you." _____

"You taste so good." _____   "Do you like it like that?" _____

"Who's your daddy?" _____   "You're the best I've ever had." _____

HERE'S WHAT I *ACTUALLY* WANT TO HEAR IN BED:

"You're *sooo* hot." _____   "Did you come yet?" _____

"Now that I've gone down on you…" _____   "I love going down on you." _____

"You taste so good." _____   "Do you like it like that?" _____

"Who's your daddy?" _____   "You're the best I've ever had." _____

WANNA DO SOME ROLE-PLAYING?

Cosmo asked women to reveal their top role-playing fantasies. See if you share their desires, and have your guy check out your thoughts on their flights of fancy. (So, whaddya say?)

FOR HER

THE STRIPPER **"Most guys find this surprising, but I want to be a stripper and have my man be a customer. There's something very voyeuristic about it. Plus, I'd never strip in real life, so it'd be fun to see what it might feel like."** *—Allison, 26*

◯ **I HAVE THIS FANTASY** ◯ **I DON'T HAVE THIS FANTASY**

WHY? _____

_____

_____

THE MODEL **"I have always thought that photographers are sexy. So I want the guy to pretend to take pictures of me as the model. The sexier the directions he gives me, the better."** *—LeAnne, 24*

◯ **I HAVE THIS FANTASY** ◯ **I DON'T HAVE THIS FANTASY**

WHY? _____

_____

THE SAUCY CHEF "Let's pretend we're two chefs getting extra creative in the kitchen, after the restaurant closes for the night." —*Candace, 31*

○ I HAVE THIS FANTASY ○ I DON'T HAVE THIS FANTASY

WHY? _____

_____

_____

THE BOSS "I want to be the boss and have my guy be the assistant that I can order around." —*Debra, 27*

○ I HAVE THIS FANTASY ○ I DON'T HAVE THIS FANTASY

WHY? _____

_____

_____

THE NURSE "It's cliché, but I love the idea of him being the doctor with me as the nurse." —*Kia, 22*

○ I HAVE THIS FANTASY ○ I DON'T HAVE THIS FANTASY

WHY? _____

_____

_____

CHAPTER 9

WHAT'S PORN GOT TO DO WITH IT?

THE SEXY TRUTH ABOUT PORN

Most guys are under the impression that women hate porn. Well, we may not love all the stuff you gravitate toward—like money shots, group sex, and weird fetishes that make you laugh as much as they turn you on—but watching a steamy flick together can be incredibly arousing.

I want you to know:

○ I'VE WATCHED PORN BEFORE

○ I HAVEN'T WATCHED IT BEFORE, BUT I WOULD

○ I'M NOT INTO PORN.

First, check out the results of a **cosmopolitan.com** poll, conducted in conjunction with **esquire.com**, to uncover the truth about how men and women today experience porn. Afterwards, each of you will get to add your own answers below each statistic. Be honest!

In a survey of 4,000 men and women between the ages of 18 to 34:

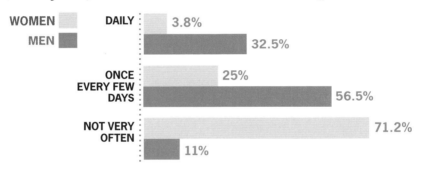

WOMEN / MEN

DAILY	3.8% (women) / 32.5% (men)
ONCE EVERY FEW DAYS	25% (women) / 56.5% (men)
NOT VERY OFTEN	71.2% (women) / 11% (men)

Here's how often I watch porn: _____
Three out of every four people surveyed said they'd watch porn with their partner.

When asked if they'd ever want to do porn or create sex tape, here's how women answered:

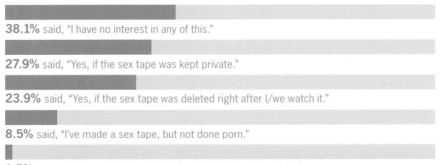

38.1% said, "I have no interest in any of this."

27.9% said, "Yes, if the sex tape was kept private."

23.9% said, "Yes, if the sex tape was deleted right after I/we watch it."

8.5% said, "I've made a sex tape, but not done porn."

1.5% said, "I'd like to try it and would be fine with it going public."

What women who were surveyed say they'd think if they found out that someone they were dating watched kinky porn:

Why doesn't he do that with me? **41.6%**

It's his private time. **35.3%**

That's fine, as long as he doesn't bring it into my bed. **20%**

I need to end this relationship now. **3.1%**

According to the men who responded to the survey, the most popular type of porn for guys is:

Who women look at when watching porn:

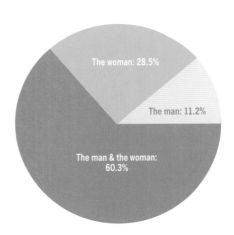

One woman: 16.4%

Two or more women: 29.4%

One man and one woman: 77.8%

Two or more men: 9.6%

The woman: 28.5%

The man: 11.2%

The man & the woman: 60.3%

- More than three in four women think women in porn are faking their orgasms.

- 14% of the women surveyed liked to watch things they wouldn't do themselves.

- 85% of the men surveyed would ask a woman to do something they've seen in porn.

Now it's your turn. You and your partner answer the following questions and share your responses with each other, to open up the dialogue on one of the hottest convos you may ever have!

| FOR HER | FOR HIM |

Have you ever watched porn before?

FOR HER
- ○ YES
- ○ NO

FOR HIM
- ○ YES
- ○ NO

Do you want to watch porn with your partner?

FOR HER
- ○ YES
- ○ NO

FOR HIM
- ○ YES
- ○ NO

Do you want to act out sex scenes from a porn movie with your partner?

FOR HER
- ○ YES
- ○ NO

FOR HIM
- ○ YES
- ○ NO

Would you ever create a sex tape?

FOR HER
- ○ YES
- ○ NO

FOR HIM
- ○ YES
- ○ NO

Do you think that women in porn are faking thier orgasms?

FOR HER
- ○ YES
- ○ NO

FOR HIM
- ○ YES
- ○ NO

What kind of porn do you like best (two women, two men, threesomes, etc?)

_____   _____

_____   _____

_____   _____

_____   _____

Let's get it out in the open: there's something I've seen in porn that I'd like to try with you, and this is what it is:

_____   _____

_____   _____

_____   _____

_____   _____

If either of your answers to any of these porn questions is "no," feel free to explain here what freaks you out about porn:

_____   _____

_____   _____

_____   _____

_____   _____

SO LET'S COME UP WITH A GAME PLAN

Cosmo has some recommendations for movies we might want to watch together. They suggest we just watch first before we step things up and mirror what we see. These porn ideas are female-friendly, which I'm sure will turn you on, too.

ANYTHING BY ERIKA LUST

This porn director makes indie flicks with realistic, chick-friendly scenarios (meaning no cheerleaders getting double-teamed by creepy dudes). They feature seriously sexy actors and plenty of sensual appeal: great music, gorgeous sets, to-die-for lingerie.

○ THESE SOUND LIKE THEY'RE WORTH A SHOT
○ I'M NOT FEELING IT ON THIS ONE

PORN FROM BRIGHTDESIRE.COM

The short films on this website include real couples having passionate, intimate, fun sex—you can tell they're truly enjoying it—and they emphasize women's Os, rather than men blowing their load. There's also a series of solo masturbation scenes, where guys pleasure themselves while describing the fantasy they're envisioning.

○ I'D LIKE TO WATCH SOME OF THESE TOGETHER
○ REAL-PEOPLE PORN DOESN'T SOUND GOOD TO ME

VIOLET BLUE

This author's women's erotica compilations are as smart as they are sexy—and female pleasure is spotlighted in every story.

○ **LET'S READ SOME OF THESE STORIES ALOUD TO EACH OTHER**

○ **NAH, LET'S PASS**

XXX PARODIES

Watch kinked-up versions of classic movies and TV shows, from *The Breakfast Club* to *Sex and the City*. Go to axxxparody.newsensations.com/home.html.

○ **THIS SOUNDS HILARIOUS, LET'S CHECK THEM OUT**

○ **SOUNDS STUPID**

THE OPENING OF MISTY BEETHOVEN

Released in 1976, this is one of the first mainstream skin flicks. It has a glam-sultry '70s vibe, and the plot is relatively interesting: A sexologist makes a bet that he can turn a low-level prostitute, Misty, into an irresistible seductress via a series of lusty lessons. Misty begins to fall for him, but the tables turn in a surprise ending. Warning: Prepare for some fuzzy hippie-era muff shots.

○ **I'M INTRIGUED—LET'S CHECK THIS OUT**

○ **"HIPPIE-ERA MUFF SHOTS"? NO THANKS**

CHAPTER 10

JUST TOYING AROUND

4 REASONS TO HAND HIM YOUR VIBRATOR

Like most men, you probably have strong opinions on whether you want to bring a vibrator into the bedroom. But a recent study shows that a majority of guys are willing to try out a buzzy toy during sex. Tell your guy, "I don't want you to be worried I'll like it better or that it'll replace you between the sheets…all it does is enhance everything for me (and, therefore, for you, too)!" We've listed the best ways to bring a vibrator into bed.

1. During oral, hold the side of the vibrator against your cheek as you lick my clitoris. It'll make your tongue quiver even more and feel unexpected and arousing for me.

   ○ **THIS SOUNDS GREAT TO ME**
   ○ **YOU CAN SKIP IT**

2. While using your mouth to pleasure me, put the vibrator inside me so it's slightly angled toward my belly button—this way, it'll hit my G-spot.

○ **THIS SOUNDS GREAT TO ME**
○ **YOU CAN SKIP IT**

3. If the vibrator is small enough, set it on low and place it between your penis and testicles during sex. The vibrations feel great against your balls, and it'll reverberate through me as you move in and out of me.

○ **THIS SOUNDS GREAT TO ME**
○ **YOU CAN SKIP IT**

4. When I'm on top, use it on my clitoris. Start with the slowest speed, and as I get more excited, turn it up to full blast.

○ **THIS SOUNDS GREAT TO ME**
○ **YOU CAN SKIP IT**

I'm most excited to try #_____ because _____

SEXY WAYS TO USE A VIBRATOR WITH HIM

Cosmo recommends turning the tables—and having you use a vibrator on him. Here are some expert tips— check them out, and each of you mark which ones you'd like to try.

Buzz it on him before you strip him down. Lay him on the bed, turn it on, and rub it over him. Start at his knees, run up his upper thighs, and circle it around the bulge in his pants. This way, he'll get comfortable with the feeling.

○ **I'M UP FOR THIS**
○ **ARE YOU UP FOR THIS?**

Start on a slow setting, and use the tip to circle your nipples and then his. As you circle, turn up the speed. Alternate between the vibrator and sucking his nipple; he should do the same to you. The back-and-forth and the heat from your lips feel amazing.

○ **I'M UP FOR THIS**
○ **ARE YOU UP FOR THIS?**

Turn it up full throttle—the shaft of a guy's penis isn't as sensitive, so he can handle it. Then move it up one side of his package and down the other. It'll stimulate his entire penis and make him extra hard.

○ **I'M UP FOR THIS**
○ **ARE YOU UP FOR THIS?**

During oral, hold the side of your vibe against your cheek as you take him in and out. Your wet, quivering mouth will feel unexpected and arousing.

○ **I'M UP FOR THIS**
○ **ARE YOU UP FOR THIS?**

Turn it on low and wrap it in your panties to lessen the sensation. Then hold the vibrator against his boys while you fondle his shaft. A guy's testicles can't take very much stimulation, so the muffled shaking is just right.

○ **I'M UP FOR THIS**
○ **ARE YOU UP FOR THIS?**

His perineum—the small patch of skin between his balls and anus—is supersensitive. Pick up a small, egg-shaped model (putting anything bigger near his booty may freak him out), and whip it out while you're on top. As you ride him, reach behind and hold it against that area.

○ **I'M UP FOR THIS**
○ **ARE YOU UP FOR THIS?**

AND MORE TOYS WE CAN PLAY WITH!

Vibrators aren't the only toys that turn women on. Check out these others below—some of them may surprise you. Let's each rate them as "hot" or "not" to see which ones we'd both like to try together.

A MASSAGE CANDLE

As these burn, the wax turns into warm massage oil. Have him drizzle a little onto your back and give you a rubdown before things really get going.

HER		HIM	
○ HOT	○ NOT	○ HOT	○ NOT

CHOCOLATE BODY PAINT

Have him brush some onto your breasts and then slowly lick it off. It's novel, which makes the entire experience seem fun and erotic.

HER		HIM	
○ HOT	○ NOT	○ HOT	○ NOT

A FULL-LENGTH MIRROR

Prop it beside the bed every once in a while. Studies suggest that when women are able to watch themselves having sex, they get more aroused than usual. (Just agree not to take any #sexselfies, okay?)

HER		HIM	
○ HOT	○ NOT	○ HOT	○ NOT

A VIBRATING RING

You probably know what this is: a ring that fits around his penis and buzzes. It's small and, as such, less intrusive than a regular vibrator. Same payoff, though: Your clitoris gets stimulated, and the vibrations feel great against his shaft.

HER		HIM	
○ HOT	○ NOT	○ HOT	○ NOT

SPOONS

Chill two metal spoons in the freezer for a couple of hours and then glide them over each other's skin. Place one against his lips, drag it down his throat and across his nipples and abs, swirl it over his genitals and inner thighs, and go all the way down to his toes. Then he can grab the other cold spoon and do the same for you.

HER		HIM	
○ HOT	○ NOT	○ HOT	○ NOT

A COMB OR HAIRBRUSH

Have him run a comb or a soft-bristled brush over your butt cheeks or use the flat side of the brush like a paddle. Or try this: Lie on your stomach and have him straddle you and give you a back massage, slowly sweeping the brush from the top of your shoulders to the backs of your thighs.

HER		HIM	
○ HOT	○ NOT	○ HOT	○ NOT

GLOVES

Slip on one leather glove and one cashmere glove. During sex, stroke his back and chest, run your fingers through his hair, or playfully swat his butt.

HER		HIM	
○ HOT	○ NOT	○ HOT	○ NOT

A TIE

Grab one of his work ties and wrap it around his eyes as a blindfold. By restricting his sense of sight, everything else you say and do to him will be intensified. Then switch.

HER		HIM	
○ HOT	○ NOT	○ HOT	○ NOT

A BEADED NECKLACE

Roll it across his lower abs and inner thighs, giving him a gentle massage. Then coil it around his penis and roll it up and down.

HER		HIM	
○ HOT	○ NOT	○ HOT	○ NOT

BOBBY PINS

First, have him use the pointy end to lightly draw circles around—but not quite touching—your headlights. As the circles get closer and closer to your nips, they'll become really erect. Use the bobby pins as mini nipple clamps to intensify your pleasure.

HER		HIM	
○ HOT	○ NOT	○ HOT	○ NOT

A PILLOWCASE

Fold it over a couple of times and tie it around his wrists. Have your way with him, and then he can return the favor.

HER		HIM	
○ HOT	○ NOT	○ HOT	○ NOT

A CASHMERE SOCK

Slip it on his erect penis, wrap your hand around his shaft, and then gently move the sock up and down—the soft texture will feel awesome against his sensitive skin.

HER		HIM	
○ HOT	○ NOT	○ HOT	○ NOT

SO, WHICH ONE DO YOU THINK IS MY FAVORITE?

_____

_____

_____

HERE'S MY ANSWER:

_____

_____

_____

AND HERE'S WHY I'M INTO IT:

_____

_____

_____

_____